About the Author ....

Disclaimer..............................

About the Book......................

Chapter 1 - Keto Basics..7
    What is the Ketogenic Diet?...7
    Difference Between A Low Carb and a Ketogenic Diet..........7
    Benefits of a Ketogenic Diet..8
    Testing on The Ketogenic Diet...12

Chapter 2 - Keto Myths Dispelled..17
    Carbohydrates are a requirement for good health 17
    You will become vitamin deficient with a low carb/ketogenic diet 18
    Ketosis is dangerous, and possibly fatal 19
    Your kidneys will be damaged on a ketogenic diet 20
    A Low Carb/Ketogenic Diet will cause Osteoporosis 20
    A Ketogenic Diet may clog your arteries and cause Heart Disease..21
    Ketogenic Diets lack essential Antioxidants and Phytochemicals 21
    Low Carb/Ketogenic Diets will cause muscle wasting.........22
    The Weight Loss from Low Carb, Ketogenic Diets is only water weight and therefore is not real......................................22
    These diets are low in fiber and therefore detrimental to your colon..23
    Low Carb, Ketogenic Diets don't work because as soon as you go off them you put the weight back on 23
    You don't need to Exercise on the Ketogenic Diet................24

Chapter 3 - Getting Started on The Ketogenic Diet..................25
    Plan #1 - Going Cold Turkey...25
    Plan #2 - Gradually Reducing Carbohydrates by A Certain Amount Per Day...26
    Plan #3 – Gradually Remove a Carbohydrate Source Per Week...26
    Plan #4 – Kickstart Ketosis with a Water Fast 27

Chapter 4 - Recommended Foods for Optimal Fat Loss..........29
    Optimal Fat Sources..29
    Optimal Protein Sources..29
    Optimal Carbohydrate Sources...30

Chapter 5 - Further Questions About the Ketogenic Diet........31

    Are Fruits Allowed on the Ketogenic Diet?...........................31
    Is the Quality of the foods Important?.................................31
    Do I need to stay on the Ketogenic Diet forever or can I move across to Paleo?...31
    Is a Ketogenic Diet safe for Kids too? 32

Chapter 6 - Introduction to Keto Blocks **33**
    Tip #1 – Misguided Information..33
    Tip #2 – Mindset..33
    Tip #3 – Dealing with Unsupportive Family and Friends......34
    Tip #4 – Unproductive Habits...34
    Tip #5 – Sleep 34
    Tip #6 – Stress 35
    Tip #7 – Mindless Eating 35
    Tip #8 – Meal Times 36
    Tip #9 – Being Prepared..36
    Tip #10 – Eating Out/Social Pressures 37

Chapter 7 - Favorite Keto Recipes **38**
    Breakfast..38
    Snacks 39
    Dinner..40
    Basics..41

Chapter 8 - Conclusion by Naturopath Jen **43**

About the Author

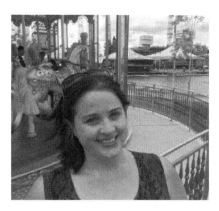

Hi there, my name is Jennifer Matthews and I am also known as Naturopath Jen. I am a qualified Naturopath, Law of Attraction Practitioner, Spiritual Life Coach and Self-Empowerment Educator. I have spent the last decade researching and spending thousands of dollars on my own personal development, as well as previously hosting multiple podcasts and blogs in the areas of health, wellness, mindset and spirituality.

I am now the founder and developer of the "Superconscious Success" Platform and the "Ask Naturopath Jen" Brand.

To learn more about myself and my journey (as it is quite an extensive read), please visit my personal site: http://www.spiritualcoachjenmatthews.com, where I delve into my purpose for writing these books and creating these brands and all the products/services (both free and paid) that can help you.

My Health Journey

Firstly, I am just like all of you. I have struggled with my own weight my entire life and after having the two children I guess I put myself last and therefore found my weight was slowly creeping up. I tried every diet imaginable prior to becoming a naturopath, I would lose a few kilograms and then of course would put it back on again. Even during naturopathic training, we are taught a lot of incorrect and outdated information and I realised this when I followed that information myself and found I was struggling.

Well, I then took it upon myself to do my own research, only to discover that a lot of what we were taught was not current and I was not being the optimal coach to my clients. I started listening to amazing podcasts and great speakers who all motivated and inspired me to not only lose my own weight but also allowed me to coach my clients to optimal health, and I have never been happier.

Following the Low Carb, Ketogenic Lifestyle has been great for me and has allowed me to lose the weight, all up until the point where I went through a stressful period in my life and I guess I fell off the band wagon (I told you I was just like you guys).

I wasn't sleeping properly, more carbs kept creeping into my diet and I lost the motivation to exercise like I once did. I knew that I felt awful, but I fell into a nonstop cascade of sugar cravings which were determined to stop me from reaching my goals.

That was until I found my hair starting to fall out, my skin starting to dry up, my memory starting to fade, and I found myself lying on the couch, unable to get up. I went to the doctor to get tested, to find out that I was diagnosed with Hashimoto's Thyroiditis, which is an autoimmune condition that attacks the thyroid gland.

Well, this may partially explain difficulty losing the weight, but I found that when I eliminated the carbs, my energy and vitality started coming back. With the power of my mind and alterations in my lifestyle I managed to kick Hashimoto's to the curb once and for all.

As a result of my current knowledge and experience with the ketogenic diet I decided to write this book in an attempt to give you the information you require to start releasing excess fat and obtain optimal health with the ketogenic diet. I am also still on a journey of discovery and I still fall off the bandwagon at times but rather than beat myself up over it, I remind myself that I am not perfect, and that today is another day.

That means that right now is what matters, the past can't be changed and the future is not determined. Try and make the right choices at this moment, little bit by little bit and praise yourself every step of the way. You will get to where you want to be if you have a strong enough desire to do so and you have the right information at your fingertips.

Disclaimer

Please note that the information given in this book is for informational purposes only and is not intended to replace the advice of your health practitioner. If you experience symptoms that you are concerned with please refer to your practitioner for further information...

About The Book

If you are wanting to lose fat, improve mental clarity and/or just improve your metabolic markers overall, then the ketogenic diet may be the perfect option for you.

After reading through multiple facebook groups and other online media, I realised that there were a couple of issues that people were struggling with the most on the ketogenic diet.

How to Get Started – They just wanted a step by step guide as to what they could and couldn't eat, the macro's they should be consuming and what to expect when they start.

What to do when they stall – Sometimes there is more going on than just the nutrition when it comes to weight loss. Although starting keto is a great way of shedding some fat, there are many other factors that can also contribute to not being as successful as what you like. I have gone briefly into 10 other things you can do to help, and the rest are covered in my next book "Keto Blocks".

So, within this guide you will find solutions to both of these problems and you can get started today...

If you would like to be notified of my upcoming books please sign up for my free membership at http://www.asknaturopathjen.com/innercircle and if you have any questions you would like answered in the next edition of the book, or you just want to give me feedback, please feel free to message me at jen@asknaturopathjen.com.

Chapter 1 - Keto Basics
****

What is the Ketogenic Diet?

The Ketogenic Diet is a Low Carb, High Fat, Moderate Protein Diet that was first introduced for the treatment of epilepsy. However, since being introduced to ketosis, a great deal of other research has been done to discover that Epilepsy is not the only condition that it treats, and that Nutritional Ketosis is remarkable when it comes to treating other conditions, including the ones that I think most people are concerned with, which is Obesity and/or Metabolic Syndrome.

Difference Between A Low Carb and a Ketogenic Diet...

There is a lot of confusion about the difference between the Ketogenic and the Low Carb Diet, but it basically comes down to the fat content and the protein content of each diet...

The Ketogenic Plan is focused on getting the body into a state of ketosis so that fat burning ability is enhanced. Fat is incredibly important when it comes to producing ketones and putting yourself into a state of ketosis and therefore the Ketogenic Diet is very high in fat (approximately 80-90%), is only moderate in protein (about 10% or so) and of course very low in carbs (<5%).

The Low Carb Diet on the other hand is more concerned with lowering the blood sugar levels, which will in turn allow you to enter fat burning mode, although possibly not as quickly as with the ketogenic diet and without the other added benefits of ketone production. This diet is not as concerned with fat or protein levels but is more focused on consuming very low carbohydrate levels to achieve this aim. Generally, the Low Carb Diet will be about 60-75% Fat, a little higher in the Protein Levels (about 20-25%) and Low in Carbs (<5%).

Benefits of a Ketogenic Diet...

There are many benefits to following the Ketogenic lifestyle.

It kills your appetite

Fat and Protein is incredibly satiating, and Carbohydrates are actually appetite stimulating, which means the Ketogenic Diet will create appetite suppression that will sometimes even make you forget to eat...

Lead to more weight loss

Due to the fact that you are producing ketones and not pumping out insulin (the fat storage hormone), you will lose fat a lot faster and a lot more efficiently than the standard weight loss diets out there...

A greater proportion of the fat will come from the abdominal region

Insulin and Cortisol are both fat storage hormones around the midsection, and when done correctly the ketogenic diet is very good at mitigating the effects of both of these hormones and ensuring that they remain balanced so that this fat is not accumulated...

Triglycerides tend to decrease

For those that don't know, triglycerides are fat molecules found in our blood and have been shown to be a contributor to heart disease. For years people thought fat consumption was going to increase triglyceride levels. However, they have since found out that it is actually only carbohydrate consumption that does this.

Increased HDL cholesterol levels

Also known as the Good Cholesterol, HDL is increased through the consumption of fats. And when I say fats, I am talking about healthy fats, and yes, I am talking about Saturated too...

Your levels of C-Reactive Protein and HbA1C will decrease

These are both markers of inflammation and heart disease risk.

Reduced Blood Sugar/Insulin Levels

Probably one of the main reasons why you would do this plan is to reduce your blood sugar levels. As sugar is toxic in the system, insulin will need to be pumped out after the consumption of carbohydrates. This insulin is then responsible for blocking the burning of fat and causing the body to store more fat. By eliminating the carbohydrates this effect will not happen.

Blood Pressure Decreases

High blood pressure (hypertension) can be a major risk factor in many diseases, but in particular heart disease. Reducing your carbohydrate levels has been shown to be an effective way of lowering your blood pressure.

Improve the pattern of LDL cholesterol

Also known as the "bad" cholesterol, for many y ears it was concluded that it was a causative factor of heart attacks and heart disease. However, now they have come to the realization that it really depends on the type of LDL cholesterol you have – Small Dense LDL (not good) or Large Fluffy LDL (not so bad). It has been shown that Low Carb and Ketogenic Diets may turn these small LDL into the large LDL and reduce the number of particles floating around in the bloodstream.

Very effective at treating various Brain Disorders

Studies have demonstrated the benefits of ketone production for treating and/or reversing many different brain disorders, such as Epilepsy, Alzheimers, ALS and even Brain Tumors. Ketones are an extremely efficient source of fuel for the brain and therefore producing them can benefit your cognition and anything else brain related considerably.

More Energy

When you are in the ketotic state you will be amazed at how much energy you have. You may find those chronic fatigue symptoms you have will have disappeared and you will be bouncing off the walls. You will be interested to know that even the slimmest person has at least 60,000 calories worth of energy on their body to tap into and therefore your level of energy is endless.

Decrease in Stiffness and Joint Pain

As this plan eliminates grains from your diet (possibly the greatest inflammatory food, alongside vegetable oils) it seems to reduce stiffness and joint pain too.

Clearer Thinking

The fogginess that tends to accompany high carb diets will disappear. As the brain is more than 60% fat, the more fat you eat the better it will be at doing its job.

Better Sleep

In most cases you will sleep better on a ketogenic diet. Of-course, there are other reasons that may prevent this from happening, which you will be able to read in my book coming up in May 2015 called The Insomniac Solution. However, generally people sleep better as the hypo-glycemia is gone, the inflammation is removed or decreased considerably and there is no longer the heartburn that comes from the inflammatory foods.

Gum Disease and Tooth Decay

Sugar is the major contributor to both of these conditions and therefore you may find that within 2-3 months on the plan any problems you have with this will decrease or disappear.

Digestion and Gut Health

As Stomach Pain, Bloating and Gas can all be associated with grain and sugar consumption, Ketogenic Diets have been shown to be effective at decreasing them.

Keto Flu...

During the first 1-4 weeks of the plan I am warning you, you may feel terrible. For those that have already gone through it you will remember the keto flu as either being something that is only mild and possibly just causes a slight headache or as something where you feel like you are going to die...

However, stick with it because I promise you, the headaches, body aches, cravings and the other symptoms you are experiencing with disappear once your body has become fully keto-adapted.

In order to avoid some of the symptoms of keto flu, it is absolutely essential that you supplement with more salt and potassium where possible. As you are losing so much water in this first 1-2 weeks you will lose a lot through the urine. Make sure you add 1 tsp of salt per day and also drink bone broth where possible.

Let me explain to you some of the reasons why you may be experiencing the keto flu:

Dizziness, Weakness and Fatigue caused by Low Blood Pressure

When you first go on a ketogenic diet, you don't end up with blood sugar spikes every time you eat. Therefore, your body is not required to pump out insulin to lower those blood glucose levels. When your insulin levels are low and stable your kidneys go into a diuretic type mode and excretes lots of sodium, potassium and water. This is why when you are first starting out, make sure you are consuming plenty of salt, water, potassium and bone broth. If you get good quality celtic sea salt that has potassium in it too.

Nausea

This will most likely happen if you go cold turkey, but I promise it won't last forever. When you consume fat, there are various pancreatic enzymes and bile salts in your liver that work to break the fats/lipids down into cholesterol, triglycerides and other components. If you start consuming more fat than your body is used to, your liver, gallbladder and pancreas don't have time to upregulate the production of bile/enzymes so as to digest this large amount of fat. This can cause you to become nauseated from the undigested fat.

Diarrhea

Alongside the point given above regarding undigested fat, there is also another reason why diarrhea will occur in the first few days. When you eat a standard diet, you consume a lot of sugar and therefore lead to the growth of non-beneficial gut flora such as Candida Albicans. Also, when we take too many antibiotics it actually kills off the beneficial bacteria in the gut making it a lot more likely that these other bacteria are going to grow. When you stop eating carbs, all of these sugar dependant bacteria die off in massive amounts and release chemicals causing temporary inflammation in the gut, therefore leading to a few days of nausea and diarrhea.

If you are new to keto, you can reduce these side effects by opting for Plan 2 or 3 of my recommended plans instead of Plan 1 or 4.

Testing on The Ketogenic Diet...

Apart from the way you are feeling, the only other way to figure out if you have entered ketosis is by testing.

There are 2 different measurements I would recommend you test for on a daily basis (if possible) when you are starting your ketogenic diet. These are Blood Glucose Levels and Ketone Levels.

Blood Glucose Levels

There is only one way to test your blood glucose levels and that is with the help of a blood glucose monitor. The good news is that blood glucose monitors and strips are actually very cheap. You are able to purchase a monitor of your choice by visiting http://www.asknaturopathjen.com/store.

There are 2 different times where I would recommend you test your blood sugar levels.

Fasting Blood Sugar levels - first thing in the morning in a fasted state.

Unfortunately, the diabetes recommendations for normal fasting blood glucose levels is too high to be really protective. Doctors will continuously tell you that under 100mg/dL (US) or 5.5 (UK/Aust) is the normal range, however the ideal range for fasting blood sugar levels is actually <86mg/dL or <4.7.

Post-Meal Blood Sugars.

There has been one test that is often given to measure your post meal blood sugars and that is the oral glucose tolerance test.

However, this is not a great test to do for a couple of reasons:

1. It is not very realistic, as not many people drink 75g of pure glucose; and
2. In people that have very poor glucose control it can be very dangerous. If you are in ketosis it can kick you out of it for a very long time.

So, instead it is recommended to get a glucometer and test your blood sugars 1-2 hours after eating.

The ADA (American Diabetics Association) recommends levels of <140/7.7 to be normal 2 hours after a meal, but these levels seem to be way too high, and can be a serious cause for concern. Research has shown that continuous levels of 140 can cause irreversible beta cell loss and nerve damage.

The majority of people's blood sugars will drop to <120 about 2 hours after a meal and then possibly even down to <100.

According to research a normal person's blood sugars 2 hours after a meal shouldn't go over 120mg/dL or 6.6.

Ketone Levels

Testing Methods

It is very important when starting the ketogenic diet that you are knowledgeable on the correct testing methods that you should be using. As each method tests for different types of ketones, it is important for you to figure out which is going to be most useful for you. If you are still looking for these devices you can get them at http://www.asknaturopathjen.com/store.

Ketostix

The most common method of testing for ketones when starting a ketogenic diet is the ketostix (pee sticks). Although these are OK to use when first starting out they are the least accurate method. They only measure the excess ketones that are being excreted via the urine and they tell you absolutely nothing about the ketones that are floating around in your blood.

Although not as accurate, these test strips are OK if you are just wanting to test how a certain food reacts with your blood sugars. They are very cheap and easy to use and as a transitional thing they seem to be alright, at least for a week or two. When I first started out on my journey I knew nothing of the other two methods of testing and it gave me an indication as to whether I was at least in some form of ketosis.

However, there are 3 main reasons you should be careful about using ketostix as a method of testing if you are really serious about succeeding on this lifestyle plan.

1. They do not measure all types of ketones in the body - Although there are 3 types of ketone bodies in our system (acetate, acetoacetate and beta-hydroxy butyrate), these strip only measure the first type - acetoacetate. When you are fully keto adapted your body may not be able to detect this form

2. of ketone (although producing substantial amounts of the others) and therefore you may get a negative result.

3. Once you are keto adapted you may excrete less ketones through the urine anyway as they are being used up and are being circulated in the blood instead.

4. Changes in hydration can also affect your concentration of ketones. Therefore, a high-water intake may dilute the concentration of the ketones in the urine, once again giving a false or a very low reading.

Blood Ketone Monitor

This is what I would consider the most accurate way of measuring whether you are in ketosis or not. The only downside however is that it is quite pricy, especially in the US. In Australia, the test strips, although not as cheap as the glucose strips are still well and truly affordable. The meter is very cheap and although it may seem scary to have to prick your finger on a daily basis it is really not that bad and is actually something that you get used to.

Although it is not absolutely necessary it is really good to be able to measure your success by testing whether you are in ketosis on a daily basis and at least with the blood ketone meter you know that it is testing for all the types of ketones. If you are not able to afford to test on a daily basis, try to get into the routine of testing at least once or twice per week to see how you are going.

Ketone levels between 1.0 and 4.0 is ideal and will indicate that you are producing a sufficient amount of the second ketone - known as Beta Hydroxybutyrate (which indicates you are burning fat).

Ketonix (Breathalizer)

This new product that has just been released is a breath tester which tests for the third type of ketone - acetone (breath). It is a one-time cost and although I believe all 3 can be beneficial at some point in your journey, the ketonix can have advantages over the other two measurement techniques:

1. As mentioned above, urine strips only test for acetoacetate and once you are actually keto adapted, this gets converted to beta hydroxybutyrate and therefore will not show up on the urine strips.

2. Urine Strips are cheap but can only be used once. The Blood Test Strips are very expensive and can only be used once. The Ketonix is only one cost (purchase of the equipment) and no strips are required. It can be used over and over again.

3. You need a bathroom to do the urine testing whereas the ketonix can be done anywhere.

Best Time Of The Day To Test

The best time of the day to test for ketones is at night, due to the fact that the level of ketones is generally lower in the morning and higher in the evening. Therefore, try to test yourself before bed to get the most accurate reading.

Chapter 2 - Keto Myths Dispelled
****

There are many myths that exist about the Ketogenic Diet and why it is supposedly dangerous for you.

Upon researching the myths that people were confronted with the most I came across an amazing website that listed 10 out of these 11 most common myths and I really want to give credit to Ellen from http://www.ketogenic-diet-resource.com for them.

She has created a website that gives plenty of resources for you to go to and look up ketogenic diets.

I have decided to give a brief overview of these myths so that I can put any doubts to rest.

If there are other myths that you are concerned about then please

let me know by emailing me at jen@asknaturopathjen.com with "myths" in the subject line so I can add it to my book.

Carbohydrates are a requirement for good health...

Well I am telling you right now, the answer is an absolute NO... The small amount of glucose that our body requires is able to be produced through other processes in the body and even the <5% of glucose in the Ketogenic Diet is sufficient to fuel the parts of the body that work best with glucose.

Every other organ in the body is very efficient at using Ketones for fuel once you are keto adapted (which can take anywhere from 1-4 weeks, depending on how glucose dependant you were in the past). The brain, in particular, loves ketones and 70-75% of its energy is able to be fueled from this source.

When you think about it, we have essential amino acids and essential fatty acids but there is no such thing as essential carbohydrates. If they were a requirement wouldn't there be a category for that...

When considering this myth, it is important to also consider people such as the Inuits and the Masai who live the ketogenic way of life.

However, I will say there is one time when carbohydrates are seen as a requirement, and that is when your body is used to consuming a high carb diet.

In this case it does not have the ability to use ketones for fuel and you will therefore find yourself entering hypo-glycemia when you get low in blood sugar.

This is why many "health experts" out there say that you should eat every 2-3 hours to avoid drops in blood sugar.

If your blood sugars were stable and your body was able to dip into your fat stores when you haven't eaten, then there would be absolutely no need to do this.

You will become vitamin deficient with a low carb/ketogenic diet...

Being one of the most common myths out there, especially by the medical establishment or the government funded dieticians, becoming vitamin deficient whilst on a ketogenic diet just does not happen.

It is important to remember that when we promote this way of eating we are promoting good quality sources that are rich in vitamins and minerals. So, let's put this myth to rest.

Firstly, people are concerned that you would be deficient in Vitamin C on this plan due to the fact that it is not recommended to eat some fruits and vegetables high in Vitamin C (such as tomatoes). What people don't know however is that you will get sufficient Vitamin C from the meat and leafy green vegetables you are going to be consuming.

Secondly, meat actually contains more vitamins and minerals than you would probably think. In fact, we could probably survive entirely on meat and fat if we had to - and some cultures actually do.

For instance, did you know that there are actually only 3 vitamins that are found in greater quantities in vegetables than in meats and that is Vitamin C, Vitamin E and Vitamin K. All the other vitamins are substantially higher in good quality animal produce - especially Vitamin B12 which is not found in vegetables.

Thirdly, when you consume the SAD diet you are generally consuming a lot of grains and legumes that are actually high in phytic acid and other anti-nutrients which bind and remove minerals from the body.

This is why when we consume high amounts of grain products in our diets, the rate of osteoporosis and other mineral disorders start to occur.

Ketosis is dangerous, and possibly fatal...

This is a concern that many people have, but the problem is that there is actually a huge difference between Ketosis and what the medical establishment is referring to, which is ketoacidosis.

Ketosis is defined as a controlled, insulin regulated process which causes a mild release of fatty acids and ketones when carbohydrates are reduced, and fats are increased.

On the other hand, Ketoacidosis is a condition that Type I Diabetics may experience when they have had a high carbohydrate meal and have not taken the required dosage of insulin. Let me explain how this situation can occur...

Type I Diabetics are not able to produce any insulin at all. Therefore, their fat calls have no insulin message telling them to hold on to fatty acids. Without this message from the insulin, a large amount of these fatty acids will flow out of the cells and be broken down into ketone bodies.

This produces an abnormally high level of ketones in the body, and as the ketones are slightly acidic in nature and there are so many floating around in the bloodstream, the blood pH will drop and cause the condition known as ketoacidosis - which is fatal.

It is important to remember that if you are producing even the littlest bit of insulin, this situation can never ever happen to you. And if you are Type I diabetic, as long as you remember to inject your insulin, this situation will not happen.

The other time that ketosis can be fatal is when you are an alcoholic and you go on a binge. This will cause a condition known as alcoholic ketoacidosis. Just remember not to binge on alcohol and you will be fine in this respect too.

Your kidneys will be damaged on a ketogenic diet...

This myth is brought about because of a misunderstanding about what a ketogenic diet really is. As long as you understand that a ketogenic diet is not a high protein diet but is actually a high FAT diet, you will understand that it will not damage your kidneys at all.

However, even if you consume a little too much protein it will NOT harm your kidneys unless you have prior kidney disease.

A Low Carb/Ketogenic Diet will cause Osteoporosis...

It has been shown that protein is actually preventative against Osteoporosis and as the ketogenic diet is moderate in protein, it will therefore lead to stronger, denser bones.

However, research has shown that magnesium deficiencies, high fructose consumption, gluten intolerance and vegetable oil consumption are all linked to osteoporosis. Well, isn't it good that these four situations don't occur on a ketogenic diet!!!

A Ketogenic Diet may clog your arteries and cause Heart Disease...

All you have to do is look at the hundreds (if not thousands) of research articles done on saturated fat and heart disease to realise that there is absolutely nothing linking cholesterol and saturated fat to cardiovascular disease.

These marketing and scare tactics have been a ploy put out by the heart association and other government bodies to scare people into taking statin drugs and other unnecessary medications.

So, do you know what it is that actually causes your arteries to clog and heart disease to follow? Carbohydrates are actually the culprit here and as elevated blood sugar and insulin levels cause inflammation in the body, it is that which has been linked to heart disease.

Studies have shown that the higher a person's HbA1c levels (marker showing a person's blood sugars for the preceding 3 months) the higher the risk of a heart attack.

Also, Insulin is a culprit when it comes to the production of cholesterol. An enzyme known as HMG-CoA is one which actually turns on the production of cholesterol in your body.

Insulin is the substance which triggers this enzyme. As insulin levels rise, so do cholesterol levels.

Ketogenic Diets lack essential Antioxidants and Phytochemicals...

Glutathione, which is our bodies naturally producing antioxidant is actually boosted by many foods commonly consumed in a ketogenic diet. Such foods include Asparagus, Broccoli, Avocado, Spinach, Eggs, Garlic and Fresh Unprocessed Meats.

Also, as mentioned previously, animal products are higher in all the vitamins and minerals than vegetables, except for 3.

Vitamin C, Vitamin K and Vitamin E were slightly lower but both Vitamin C and Vitamin K are found in the Leafy Green Vegetables and Vitamin E is found in nuts.

Did you know, that the more carbohydrates you eat, the more vitamin C you need to consume. This is due to the fact that both carbohydrates and vitamin C compete for the same metabolic pathways.

Therefore, by reducing your carbohydrates you will be able to get sufficient Vitamin C from the animal products you consume.

Low Carb/Ketogenic Diets will cause muscle wasting...

Actually, the opposite has actually been shown to be true. Studies have actually shown that ketogenic diets have a muscle sparing effect.

This myth comes from the fitness industry and personal trainers alike who say that if you don't get a certain amount of carbohydrates per day then your body will break down protein to get it.

However, this only applies if you are not keto adapted. If you are keto-adapted your body will just produce ketones to fuel other functions in the body.

As the ketogenic diet has sufficient protein in it (and probably more than the SAD diet), as well as optimal ketone production, it causes growth of lean muscle mass.

The Weight Loss from Low Carb, Ketogenic Diets is only water weight and therefore is not real...

In the first week or so of a Ketogenic Diet you will lose a lot of water. There are a few reasons for this. Firstly, as explained above, when you cut carbohydrates, blood sugar and insulin levels will come down and therefore the kidneys will dump excess water and sodium from the body.

Also, when you first start the ketogenic diet your glycogen stores will be reduced and as glycogen contains a lot of water that will also be dumped. However, as you become keto-adapted this water loss will be stabilized and the fat that you are losing is just that, fat...

Make sure when going through this first week or so that you get plenty of salt and minerals to replace the ones lost in the bathroom (ie you need to consume more salt and potassium on a ketogenic diet).

These diets are low in fiber and therefore detrimental to your colon...

Ketogenic Diets do actually promote eating plenty of green leafy vegetables, thereby making this myth absolutely false. It has been shown that people consuming a ketogenic diet actually eat more fibrous vegetables than those on a SAD diet, so eat up those vegges.

Low Carb, Ketogenic Diets don't work because as soon as you go off them you put the weight back on...

Just like with any diet if you do not continue with it over the long term, of course the weight is going to come back on. When I talk about the ketogenic diet I am talking about a change in lifestyle and a change in eating habits.

It must become a way of life for you to maintain consistent and lifelong weight loss and weight maintenance.

It is not just a plan to use while you lose the weight and then expect you can go off it and everything will stay the same. It is important to commit to it for the long term...

You don't need to Exercise on the Ketogenic Diet...

Although it is not absolutely essential to exercise on a ketogenic diet and you can lose fat without it, you will lose it much quicker if you do integrate fitness into your daily routine.

However, I do not recommend a great deal of long, slow cardio but instead recommend you include HIIT and Strength Training, along with some great stretching routines.

Please note that when you are first becoming keto adapted you may not have the energy to do some heavy exercise, so just make sure that you are at least doing some walking and integrating movement as much as you can.

I ask that you refrain from sitting too much as excessive sitting has been linked to increases in the rates of heart disease and heart attacks (amongst other ailments) and if you do need to sit for many hours a day, make sure it is doing something productive and also try to get up every 30-60 minutes and move around. You will feel a lot better doing so.

Once you feel you have the energy required for a more intensive exercise program then start to implement HIIT and Strength Training.

Chapter 3 - Getting Started On The Ketogenic Diet
****

If you are not yet on the ketogenic diet but have decided after reading the benefits that you are really interested in starting it yourself, then I will give you some basic pointers as to how to get started. Please note there are 4 different plans you can choose from when you are starting the ketogenic diet:

Plan #1 - Going Cold Turkey

Generally, this is the plan I would recommend for most people as it gets you the results the quickest. However, it is definitely tough and it will generally be a sure-fire way of having to deal with the keto flu. Plans #2 and #3 are not as strict and therefore will minimise this flu.

1. Eliminate all carbohydrates from your diet, except for leafy green vegetables. Although I don't count calories I like to keep the carbohydrates to no more than 5% of my intake.

2. Reduce your protein to about 10-15% of your calories (this number can change depending on your exercise level, your individual biology and how sensitive you are to gluconeogenesis. Although it is the number I use, you will need to readjust if it doesn't work for you).

3. Increase your fat content to approximately 80% of your calories. Although I know you can get results from a ketogenic diet with 60% of your calories from fat, I like to keep it around 80% because that means I do not get too many carbohydrates or protein in my day. However, on exercise days I may increase my protein a little and therefore end up with about 70% - 75% fat instead. Just keep tweaking it and see what works for you so that you are still producing ketones.

4. Make sure you test regularly for ketones and blood sugars. As the ketone strips can be very expensive you may only be able to test these once or twice a week. But at least you will be able to get an idea as to how they are going. I would probably start testing within a week of starting the plan to make sure that you are keto adapted.

Plan #2 - Gradually Reducing Carbohydrates By A Certain Amount Per Day

By doing this you would gradually reduce your carbohydrate levels by about 10g per day until you get down to the 20g total limit. This could take a while – especially if you are consuming a very high carb diet but it is a gentler approach that may not be as stressful mentally as the "Cold Turkey" approach.

However, make sure that you are also upping the fat intake until you reach satiety. "Do NOT increase the protein intake instead, otherwise it will just take you a bit longer to reach ketosis".

I would recommend you don't start testing for ketones until you have been down to about 30g of carbs for a whole week or 2. However I would recommend you testing blood glucose levels.

Plan #3 – Gradually Remove a Carbohydrate Source Per Week

This plan is also a gentler approach and is a lot easier than going cold turkey. It allows you to change certain habits, and because of this do like this way of doing it. However, it is important to understand that it is still not as effective as going Cold Turkey and will take a lot longer to go into ketosis.

A good example of doing this would be:

1. Week 1 – Cut out sugary sodas and replace with sugar free sodas. (However, make sure that you intend to cut those out too as they can still cause a spike in blood sugars.)

2. Week 2 – Cut out biscuits with your nighttime cup of tea;
3. Week 3 – Cut out sugary desserts and snacks;
4. Week 4 – Cut out all starches;
5. Week 5 – etc etc etc...

Keep doing this until you are down to less than 30g per day. Make sure you are upping the fat at the same time (once you get below 100g of carbs per day) and as with the plan above, moderate the protein!!!

As with Step #2 I would not recommend testing ketones until you have been under 30g for a full week or two.

Plan #4 – Kickstart Ketosis with a Water Fast

I know there is a lot of controversy about water fasting and it is certainly not for everybody, but from personal experience and after hours and hours of research I have realised that it is a great way of really getting yourself into ketosis quickly and I have had nothing but a great experience with it.

If you have plateaued or are really wanting to kickstart your ketosis quickly, you can do a water fast beforehand for a couple of days. Women tend to take about 2 days to enter ketosis after a water fast and men generally about 3 days.

I love this way of doing it and not only is it great to help you enter ketosis but there are also so many added benefits to it.

Please note that you will most likely still experience symptoms of the keto flu (especially the low blood pressure and some diarrhea due to the bacteria being eliminated) so make however that if you are going to do this that you eat really clean (vegetables, good quality meat etc) for at least a few days beforehand so the body doesn't get too shocked, and make sure you consume some celtic sea salt at the same time so as to minimize the effects of the blood pressure.

Note that when you go to increase your fats afterwards you may still experience the nausea and diarrhea due to the high fat content but it shouldn't be as bad as the fasting would have removed all the negative bacteria anyway.

Once you have done the fast, then go cold turkey...

If you have a pre-existing condition, please check with your health practitioner first to see if it would be OK.

Chapter 4 - Recommended Foods For Optimal Fat Loss
****

Optimal Fat Sources

1. Butter
2. Ghee
3. Lard
4. Tallow
5. Sour Cream
6. Heavy Cream
7. Double Cream
8. Full Fat Cheese
9. Olives
10. Avocado
11. Bacon
12. Coconut Oil
13. Duck Fat

Optimal Protein Sources

High Fat Beef Cuts (from highest in fat to lowest) - Rib Eye Steak, T-Bone Steak, New York Strip Steak, Skirt Steak, Porterhouse Steak, Filet Mignon, Flap Steak, Top Sirloin, Bottom Round, Eye of Round Steak, Top Round Steak, Sirloin Tip Side Steak. - Choose the high fat cuts if you are eating grass fed beef, or low fat if eating conventional beef.

High Fat Poultry Cuts (all free range where possible and limited as it is high in omega 6 fats) - Chicken Skin, Chicken wing with skin, Chicken thigh with skin, Duck, Goose, Chicken drumstick with skin, Chicken breast with skin.

High Fat Fish (high in omega 3 fat and low in mercury) - Anchovies, Herring, Mackerel (Canned), Oysters, Salmon (Canned or Fresh), Sardines, Trout.

Free Range Eggs.

Optimal Carbohydrate Sources

Pretty much the only carbohydrate you will consume on the Ketogenic Diet will be vegetables. Therefore, there are many vegetables you can still enjoy on a ketogenic diet.

I have included approximate counts of the top 25 vegetables I consume on this plan, which are all 2g or less per 1/2 cup.

1. Mustard Greens - 0.1 per 1/2 cup
2. Chopped Parsley - 0.1 per 1/2 cup
3. Raw Spinach - 0.1 per 1/2 cup
4. Bok Choy - 0.2 per 1/2 cup
5. Endive - 0.2 per 1/2 cup
6. Lettuce (Iceberg) - 0.2 per 1/2 cup
7. Lettuce (Romaine) - 0.2 per 1/2 cup
8. Alfalfa Sprouts - 0.2 per 1/2 cup
9. Turnip Greens (Boiled) - 0.6 per 1/2 cup
10. Raddichio - 0.7 per 1/2 cup
11. Broccoli Florets - 0.8 per 1/2 cup
12. Cauliflower (Steamed) - 0.9 per 1/2 cup
13. Garlic Clove (Fresh) - 0.9 per clove
14. Radishes - 0.9 for 10
15. Raw Cucumber - 1 per 1/2 cup
16. Jalapeno Peppers - 1 per 1/2 cup
17. Green Raw Cabbage - 1.1 per 1/2 cup
18. Cooked Shiitake Mushroom - 1.1 per 1/2 cup
19. Summer Squash - 1.3 per 1/2 cup
20. Red Raw Cabbage - 1.4 per 1/2 cup
21. Raw Cauliflower - 1.4 per 1/2 cup
22. Button Mushrooms - 1.4 per 1/2 cup
23. Zucchini (Steamed) - 1.5 per 1/2 cup
24. Steamed Asparagus - 1.6 for 4 Spears
25. Steamed Green Cabbage - 1.6 per 1/2 cup

Chapter 5 - Further Questions About The Ketogenic Diet
****

Are Fruits Allowed on the Ketogenic Diet?

As the carbohydrate allowance is so low, it is very likely you will not be able to eat any fruit to begin with. Over time as you become more insulin sensitive you may be able to include berries with heavy whipping cream (and possibly even some dark chocolate) to your regime.

Is the Quality of the foods Important?

I have always believed that the quality of food is of utmost importance, in terms of it being locally grown, organic, grass fed and raw.

It should be in its unaltered state where it could almost be pulled from the ground and eaten in the state it is in. However, I have a caveat to this.

If you do not have the funds to source grass fed beef or organic vegetables, then that is OK. It is much better to at least start off by implementing the Ketogenic Macronutrient Ratios and then one step at a time improve the quality of it.

Do I need to stay on the Ketogenic Diet forever or can I move across to Paleo?

I am an absolute massive fan of the Paleo/Primal Plans and once you are insulin sensitive and you have lost the weight you are wanting to lose, and assuming you don't have any brain disorders you are wanting to heal, then of course it is perfectly fine to convert from Ketogenic to Paleo.

The Ketogenic Diet may not be necessary for everybody and it certainly may not be necessary for you to do for the rest of your life. However, there is no reason you can't. I plan on living this lifestyle for as long as I possibly can as I absolutely love the effects from the plan itself, so I can't see myself changing anytime soon.

Don't allow anybody to pressure you into changing your way of eating if it is making you feel good and all your markers are looking good too...

Is a Ketogenic Diet safe for Kids too?

A Ketogenic Diet is absolutely safe for kids and it has been shown to help their cognitive performance. Remember that it will take a little while for them to convert to fat burning which means they may get the symptoms of the keto flu to start with.

Because of this I would recommend you transition them during school holidays and not during the school term when mental acuity must be at its peak...

Chapter 6 - Introduction to Keto Blocks
****

If you have managed to do everything here but you are still struggling to lose weight, how about you check out my first 10 keto blocks that may be halting you from keto success.

For further details on these or to get even more tips (once you have altered these and still don't have the success you are looking for), keep an eye out for my other book "Keto Blocks".

However, the first 10 I am going to suggest are as follows:

Tip #1 – Misguided Information

Make sure that you are following a plan that is right for you and that you check up on it if something does not sound quite right.

If you are not sure about the plan you are going to be following then you may end up only doing half the plan (as is shown in people doing a low fat, low carb diet because they think if only they have low fat as well, they are bound to lose the weight).

Tip #2 – Mindset

Although this is a massive topic that will be detailed in greater detail in my next book, it is incredibly important that you make sure you have a positive mindset when embarking on a new weight loss / health venture.

If you have a negative mindset it will be a lot easier to fall of track and be unable to get back on. By being positive you can train your mind through visualizations and affirmations to help progress you towards the goals you are looking for.

Tip #3 – Dealing with Unsupportive Family and Friends

This is possibly one of the biggest problems I found people were having with their own journey and so it is one I have gone into with great detail.

However, one point I am going to make here is that all you can do is educate your loved ones about why you are doing it and show them the progress you are making.

If you end up around family and/or friends that are always negative, try to dissociate yourself from them and learn to switch off when they begin to be negative.

It is important to remember that you can't change somebody that doesn't want to be changed and you can't make somebody support you if you are not yet ready to do so.

Tip #4 – Unproductive Habits

Now I want you to take a look at your lifestyle and notice habits that may be hindering your success. This could be that daily cappuccino you are consuming or that partying you are doing on the weekend. Once you acknowledge these habits, make changes in your lifestyle to replace them with more positive ones.

Tip #5 – Sleep

This is absolutely critical. Without good quality sleep you will be pumping out hormones that are not beneficial and you will be stopping the hormones that are required for weight loss.

For this step try to get your circadian rhythm in check by going to bed at the same time every night and getting up at the same time every morning.

Tip #6 – Stress

Learn to manage your stress levels. With our busy lives and trying to juggle many things at once, stress has become a normal part of everyday life.

I even think that people don't recognise that they are stressed anymore. Because of this, our adrenals are constantly depleted, and our system is pumping out hormones like cortisol, which are fat storing hormones.

With this step I would like you to start by learning deep breathing techniques and possibly meditation or self-hypnosis.

Tip #7 – Mindless Eating

Our society has gotten so used to eating on the run or sitting in front of the television and eating that we don't even know what we are eating half the time.

We forget to chew properly because we aren't focusing and then within 5 minutes the meal is gone, and our stomach is still signalling that we are hungry.

By making sure that you are mindful when you are eating you give your body time to realize that it is full and therefore you end up eating a lot less. You also enjoy your meal a lot more because you are able to actually taste and focus on what you are able to put in your mouth.

With this step I would like you to first make sure you sit at a table for a meal without any television or radio on and just focus on the meal you are eating.

Count the chews if you can (that is what I do) and you will be surprised how much less you eat. Also, make sure that you eat in an unstressed state where possible because when you are stressed it puts a stop to digestion and therefore you will not be absorbing all the nutrients required.

If you are looking for a great book to teach you about eating mindfully, then get "French Women Don't Get Fat" from my store at http://www.asknaturopathjen.com/store or visit Amazon and get your copy.

Tip #8 – Meal Times

Although when you eat is not necessarily as important as what you eat it can still be a problem if you are eating the largest portion of calories later on in the day as it means you are going to bed on a full stomach.

It is much preferable to have your breakfast or lunch meal as your main meal and then a lighter snack at night time. I like to make sure that my breakfast and lunch meals are high fat, high protein and my dinner meal more of a salad with a small amount of protein.

The reason for this is because it means I am burning as much fat as I can around breakfast and lunch as there are no carbs in that meal.

The night-time carbs are used overnight and so you will be back in a fasting state when you wake up. Try it out. You will notice a difference.

Tip #9 – Being Prepared

When I talk about being prepared, I mean both mentally and physically. When it comes to being mentally prepared you need to be aware about what the keto diet is and what symptoms you are most likely going to experience with the keto flu, as well as be prepared in case any cravings come up.

The other interesting thing you need to be prepared for is the fact that you will not be very hungry on this plan and may have to force yourself to eat. Some people can get very worried when they lose their appetite, so it is important for you to understand you may lose your appetite on this plan.

You also need to be physically prepared by cleaning out the pantry, fridge and freezer so you are not tempted to dig into those old staples.

Tip #10 – Eating Out/Social Pressures

This is another big one that people have issues with. What do you do when you go out to eat or when you are at somebody's house and you don't want to offend them.

I would recommend during the first two weeks of the program when you are becoming fat adapted that you avoid eating out as much as possible and that way you can control what you are putting into your mouth.

After that time it is important to learn to choose foods that are as close to fitting in your plan as possible. However, try to refrain from eating fast foods too often as these frankenfoods are not beneficial to your success.

Before going to a party or to somebody's house eat something beforehand so you are not hungry when you get there. If you have to, tell them that you are celiac or gluten intolerant and that will at least eliminate the grainy products and then go from there.

So, these are my first 10 keto blocks which are found in greater detail in my upcoming book "Keto Blocks". If you are struggling with losing weight on the ketogenic diet then these blocks are your first step.

Chapter 7 - Favorite Keto Recipes

****

Breakfast

Keto Eggs

One of my favorite keto meals is of course eggs. However to bring it up to Keto macronutrient standards you also have to make sure that you include a lot of fat with it.

Therefore, I like to eat scrambled eggs with added fat. Put some bacon on the side and some spinach cooked in homemade lard and you have an awesome meal.

Ingredients Include:

3 Eggs
1/8 cup Heavy Cream
1 tsp Celtic Sea Salt
1 Tbsp Sour Cream
1/4 Avocado
1 Tbsp Coconut Oil
2 Strips Bacon
100g Spinach fried in 1/2 tbsp Lard

Method:

Firstly, you need to mix the eggs with the heavy cream and 1 tsp celtic sea salt. Scramble it up in the coconut oil so that the yolks are still slightly runny but the whites are cooked. Chop up the avocado into small pieces and add that and the sour cream on top of the eggs. Put this alongside the bacon and spinach and you have a great keto meal.

Snacks

Snack #1 - Keto Bomb - Cinnamon Fat Bomb

One of my favorite snacks of all times - which I know are keto friendly are fat bombs. There are so many out there... All you need to do is go to pinterest and you will find so many, depending on what foods you are wanting to include.

However, my favorite fat bomb ever is the following:

Ingredients Include:

1 cup Coconut Butter
1 cup Coconut Milk (try to get milk that does not have BPA in the can)
1 cup Shredded Coconut
1 tsp Vanilla Extract
1/2 tsp Nutmeg
1/2 tsp Cinnamon
2 tsp Sweetner of your Choice

Method:

1. Melt the Coconut Butter, Coconut Milk, Vanilla Extract, Nutmeg, Cinnamon and Sweetener in a double broiler over medium heat. If you don't have a double broiler, place it in a metal bowl inside of a pan with some water in it.
2. Make sure you continue to mix the ingredients as they melt.
3. Pour in the Shredded Coconut and mix up.
4. Place into moulds and put in the fridge. You can also roll into balls instead if you like.
5. Refrigerate for 1 to 2 hours or even place in the freezer as a nice frozen snack on a hot day.

Snack #2 - Keto Creamsicle

Ingredients Include:

1 cup Heavy Whipping Cream

2-3 tsp Sweetener of Choice (adjust the sweetener depending on your preference and depending on how many you are making) 1/2 tsp Raw Cocoa Powder
1 tsp Vanilla Extract
1/2 tsp Cinnamon

Method:

1. Mix together all ingredients.
2. Place into a popsicle mould.
3. Freeze.

Dinner

It is important to understand that meals don't have to be tricky to make or really complicated to be good for you. I love meals that are quick and easy and yet incredibly tasty. Because of that I have decided to include my favorite keto dish - which is really delicious but also incredibly nutritious.

Poached Salmon with Coconut Cream

Ingredients Include:

1 medium piece of salmon, with skin on (wild caught if possible);
1 tsp turmeric
1 clove garlic
1 cup coconut cream (in a BPA free can where possible)
Ketogenic Vegetables of Choice (no more than 3) cooked in your fa of choice.

Method:

1. Place the piece of salmon into a skillet.
2. Pour in the coconut cream, turmeric and garlic.
3. Simmer over medium heat for no more than 5 minutes on the first side and 2-3 minutes on the second side (depending on how well-done you like your salmon).
4. Put with your keto vegetables.
5. Enjoy.

Basics

One of the best fats you could possibly eat when on a ketogenic diet is that of lard. So I thought the fifth recipe for me to include would be how to render down your own homemade Lard (and believe me it tastes really good...)

Rendering Lard

Methods Include:

1. Go to your local butcher and ask for 4-5 lbs of leaf lard if possible (fat from around the kidneys of the pig).
2. Cut or grind this fat into small pieces. Often it is much easier to do if you have allowed it to harden up a little in the freezer (not completely freeze it though).
3. Add 1/4 cup of water to the bottom of a crockpot and add the cut-up pork fat.
4. Set the crockpot to low and let it go for about an hour. Keep checking to make sure that the fat is not burning. When the fat begins to melt it will separate itself from the crackling. When this happens (about 1.5 - 2 hours in) the cracklings will settle at the bottom and the fat is ready to start being separated.
5. Ladle this fat through some cheesecloth so as to separate the fat from the crackling.
6. At this point the cracklings will still be soft and not crispy.
7. Ladle this fat into mason jars. The fat will look yellow or white (if using leaf lard).
8. Let the fat cool on the counter.

9. Store in the refrigerator or freezer.
10. Return the cracklings to the crockpot and allow it to keep going until it is crispy. Add these to salads.
11. Remember that it could take 4-5 hours to complete the process entirely, depending on how much fat you are using. But it is definitely worth it...

Chapter 8 - Conclusion By Naturopath Jen
****

I hope that you have received all the information you need from this Book to really get started on your own journey. If you are looking for the next step up from this book, then my advanced manual Keto Blocks is also for sale.

Keto Blocks goes through 40 reasons why you may be plateauing on your weight loss journey and includes such topics as mindset, sleep, stress, environment, nutrition, fitness, thyroid and much much more...

To get access to this book you can go to http://www.asknaturopathjen.com/store.

Aside from that, please go to my website and sign up for my FREE Inner Circle Membership at http://www.asknaturopathjen.com/innercircle. You will then receive notification once the other books are out as well as a variety of information on ketosis. On top of that I ask that you please rate and review this book on Amazon, so it may reach more and more people. I really appreciate it.

Cheers
Naturopath Jen

Made in the USA
Las Vegas, NV
13 January 2022

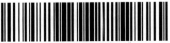